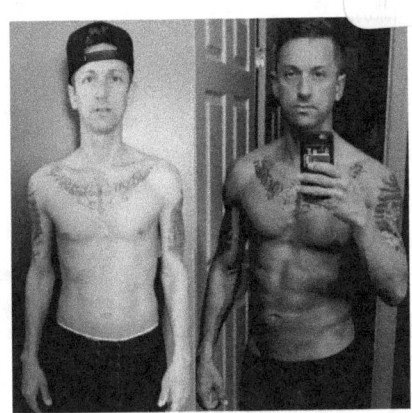

The Testosterone Solution

Dr. Tammy Post

BetterLiving **RX**

Live Better Longer

ISBN-13: 978-1540771933
ISBN-10: 1540771938

DEDICATION

To my husband who inspires me to create and supports me everyday to spread the mission of helping others live their best lives possible. His commitment to empowering others through balancing their health is unstoppable. He's a beast! (I'd take credit for his tenacity in spreading this message but it's probably due to the "T", LOL)

I love you, honey!

WARNING

If you don't know if this book is for you... or if you think low "T" Testosterone couldn't possibly affect you then please skip ahead to chapter 2!

TABLE OF CONTENTS

ACKNOWLEDGMENTS

To Jeremy and Jill Jones for taking our mission forward and the use of their beautiful photos for this book.
To all our coaches who make hormone balance possible for the masses and demystify the phony science everyday and bring others the opportunity to be at their very best.
To our staff and families who sacrifice and support us always.
To you out there who have struggled and to those who support the empowered health of men and women everywhere.

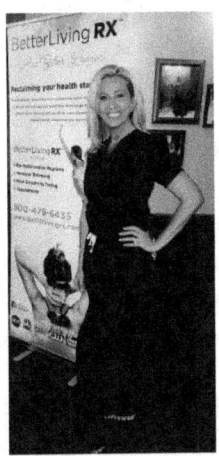

Introduction
WHO AM I?

You may be wondering...

Who am I and why should you listen to me?

I am a board-certified family physician who left the rat race of traditional medicine to help others find balance and reclaim their youth and vitality. Why?

Because I have struggled in many areas related to hormone balance. Through my own journey of female hormone issues, weight gain, debilitating pain from inflammation, and chronic fatigue, I began helping others in ways that traditional medicine had absolutely no answers for. Traditional medicine is driven by the pharmaceutical and insurance companies. This realization became clear to me during my freshman year in medical school. I was feeling overwhelmed when a very kind and well-meaning professor took me aside in class one day and whispered, "Don't worry, Tammy...you'll memorize a handful of medications used to treat the most common illnesses and that will be all you really need to know to make a good living as a doctor. Just survive and pass the tests. Trust me..."

At first this sounded like the grand relief I had been looking for and exactly what I wanted and needed to hear. I took a deep breath. Part of me was saying, "Really?!?!? That's awesome!" The other part of me was thinking, "What the Hell???? Are you kidding me? That's horrible!" But over the years I have learned just how true that statement is today. I'm not saying that your doctors don't care or that they have any ill intent. I am saying that we are taught a way that is built upon the early doctors of the 18th century: Poisoning people with medications and chemo, using radiation, and cutting out vital organs. We have lost our connection to true physiology and its applicability to our health and ongoing youth and vitality.

We are offered pharmaceuticals for every ill. I call it a "pill for an ill", which has been suspended forever on this merry-go-round we call medical care in the U.S. **Now my disclaimer here is not to fire your doctor or quit any medication.** What I am saying is that you need to step up, take full responsibility for your health, and empower yourself to take the steps necessary to reclaim your health, youth, and vitality.

A Story About Cholesterol

When I was in residency for my family medicine training, I had another interesting glimpse in to the world of pharmaceuticals. I was invited to one of the nicest restaurants in town to hear a pretty little drug rep give a lecture on the benefits of cholesterol-lowering medication. Before she finished she said something that absolutely terrified me. She said that if I have a patient with even borderline high cholesterol and I don't put them on this medication, they could sue me. As a new doctor who had not yet made her first dollar this was more than just unsettling. If what she said was true, a patient could sue me before I even began earning a living simply for not putting them on a drug.

The next day I went to my training space (as a resident this was basically a small cubicle) and looked up everyone for which I had done cholesterol level screens. I then instructed my nurse to call each one and get them on this drug right away.

And so for years I practiced fear-based medicine. Sadly, this is standard practice with so many doctors to this day.

You see, the truth is we think that cholesterol is just a glob of grease sitting in our arteries waiting to cause a heart attack or stroke and kill us.

Not true. Cholesterol is a hormone made by the liver (approximately 80%) to create all our other essential sex hormones (like testosterone, estrogen, and even cortisol) through enzymatic conversions.

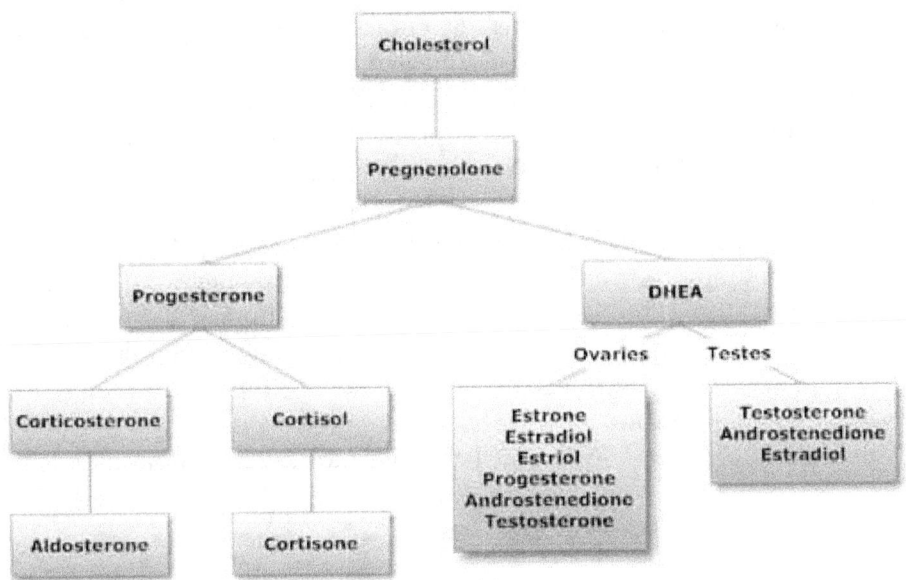

We need our cholesterol! The sneaky thing is the pharmaceutical companies are tickled pink when we suppress cholesterol because without those other hormones we get sick, age, and feel terrible very quickly. And they sell lots of drugs for those ills.

This is not a discussion on cholesterol so I won't go into the fact that thousands of studies have shown that most people who have suffered heart attacks and strokes have 'normal' cholesterol levels. Furthermore, that inflammation caused by hormone imbalance is one of the major culprits.

I will say to you that you should be aware and never assume or blindly take medication of any kind without first asking some serious questions.

Over the past 16 years I have treated an estimated 30,000 men and women and I have found that the answers are usually quite simple.

It's not one thing that causes us to get out of balance and it's not one thing that fixes it. There are no magic pills or quick fixes that will restore your health, youth, and vitality. What is required is your commitment to empowering yourself with knowledge and some dedication to making some healthy choices to support your beliefs.

I started out treating mostly women because our hormone issues and physiology are so diverse and complicated. If I could tap into my own journey, I knew I could better understand how to offer some relief. Understandably, many of the women who had started feeling amazing wanted their husbands to feel as good as they did. When we restored libido or gave them one for the first time they wanted their partners to 'catch up'! I always tell women two things: Testosterone can make you want someone but not 'like' them (and then they laugh); and men's issues are easily fixed most of the time with just restoring testosterone levels, while women have a more complicated milieu of hormones which can affect our moods and emotions.

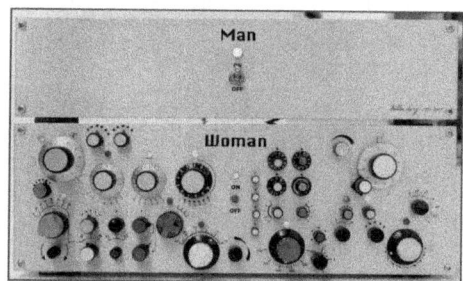

Ladies, if you are reading this for your man we have answers for you too. And men, if you are reading this I hope that you will start to get a glimpse of how freaking lucky you are to have such a simple solution:

THE TESTOSTERONE SOLUTION.

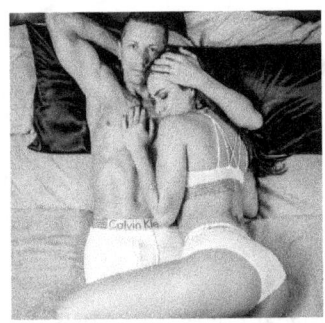

CHAPTER 1 - IS THIS FOR ME?

"My testosterone is fine!" is what I frequently hear from guys who will defend their serum testosterone levels like they would their very manhood, reputation, or family name.

The truth is that if you are a male over the age of 30 it's probably not what you think it is. You know deep down that you can't go play football with the teenagers like you used to without getting injured easily. You don't have the stamina that you did at 17, you get tired, and need to take a nap when you get home from work. You don't have the drive you used to have that got things done. Or maybe you have gained weight in the belly.

Maybe you have one of the following:

☐ Bad moods or irritability/sadness
☐ Weight gain
☐ Muscle loss
☐ Mental, emotional, physical sluggishness
☐ Decrease in sex drive
☐ Inadequate erections
☐ Poor sleep
☐ Lack of strength and endurance
☐ Difficulty focusing
☐ A lack of joy for life and living

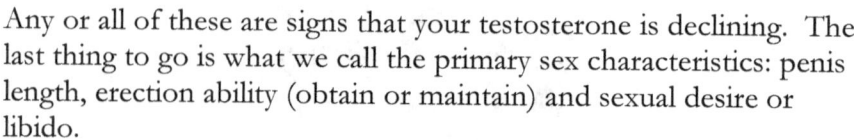

Any or all of these are signs that your testosterone is declining. The last thing to go is what we call the primary sex characteristics: penis length, erection ability (obtain or maintain) and sexual desire or libido.

Does This Sound Like Your Story? As a man, can you identify with any of the following?

☐ You used to have tons of energy, but now you always feel exhausted ... and you can't remember the last time you had a good night of sleep.

☐ You get those mystery aches and pains that seem to show up out of the blue.

☐ You have muscle loss and have gained weight ... even if you are working out as hard as you used to.

☐ You have trouble concentrating or focusing on even the easiest tasks ... remembering the simplest things can be a struggle.

☐ You find yourself feeling sad, moody, irritable, or down ... even when everything on the outside appears to be okay.

☐ You don't have the "get up and go" like you used to in the bedroom ... your sex drive and ability falling by the wayside.

This isn't the way it was supposed to happen, is it?

You used to feel like a man, but now you are left to talk about things like erectile dysfunction, poor sex drive, and lack of energy with your doctor.

It's frustrating and embarrassing, isn't it?

Whether the changes happened gradually or they happened overnight, you want your life back and you want it back ASAP.

When my patients ask me, "How did I get like this?" I tell them, "It's like boiling a frog.

You boil a frog by putting him in cold water and slowly turn up the heat. It's so gradual the frog doesn't realize it's cooked till it's cooked!" And so it goes with hormone imbalance. It's slow and gradual till you find you feel bad or maybe you don't even realize how bad you feel because it was so gradual. It's what I describe to my patients as your 'new normal'.

One night my husband and I were eating out and we watched gentlemen with their wives going into the restaurant. I have been treating men with low testosterone, or "Low T" as we call it for short, for many. I have come to know just by guessing their age and how overweight they are what their testosterone levels are. I'm pretty spot on after all this time.

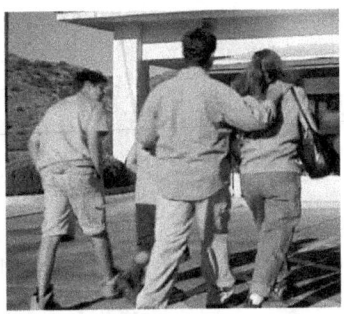

Because the enzyme aromatase is stored in fat cells, for every pant size you are overweight you have about 33% more aromatase. This aromatase converts your testosterone to estrogen.

Testosterone   Estradiol

This lowers your testosterone which causes your testicles to shrink and your breasts to enlarge ('man boobs'.) You can feel depressed, tired, and not your best. Because you are tired you don't pursue fitness opportunities, causing you to gain more weight and the cycle just worsens.

Let's have a little fun. Would you like to know what your levels are approximately without a blood test?

Let me give you a little history. I read about this study from the British Medical Journal that showed an increased risk of breast cancer of 33% per skirt size that a person goes up after menopause. I asked "what causes this increase?" And the obvious answer was increase in aromatase enzyme, the enzyme that converts testosterone to estrogen metabolites (namely, estrone-the proliferative estrogen) and realized that this reduction in testosterone is significant and translate to me to increased estrogens and therefore more weight gain and risk of prostate (proliferative) type cancers. Through my clinical experience and my disclaimer here, I will tell you that interestingly this 33% correlates perfectly to the decrease in testosterone with andropause related weight gain. Also, if you are not overweight, don't stop reading now because there are many other factors which can reduce testosterone (genetics, environmental, nutritional deficiencies like zinc and selenium, thyroid or other hormone imbalances and alcohol due to inappropriate clearance through the liver. In fact some studies have shown almost a 33% correlation in reduced testosterone just as impactful as being overweight, so you could do the estimation based on how much alcohol you drink, potentially. A good reason to cut out the booze. ☺

New Study: Increase in Skirt Sizes Increases

Risk of Breast Cancer

Going up several skirt sizes in midlife could be a warning sign of increased cancer risk, research suggests.

According to a new study published in the British Medical Journal, increasing your skirt size with each decade could raise the risk of breast cancer by one third.

The study by the University College London of more than 90,000 women found that those whose skirt size went up for each decade between their twenties and sixties increased their risk of developing breast cancer after the menopause by 33%. Further, women whose size increased by two regardless of their overall weight in the same period saw an increased risk of a whopping 77%. The women were all aged over 50, had gone through the menopause, and had no known breast cancer when they entered the study between 2005 and 2010.

While obesity has long been known to increase the risk of cancers, there is growing evidence to suggest that a thickening of the waist holds specific dangers.

Researchers said extra fat on the waist may boost levels of estrogen in the body, which increases the risk of breast cancer. After taking account of other influential factors, increases in skirt size emerged as the strongest predictor of breast cancer risk.

So here's the formula (and again this is just an extrapolation based on my clinical experience that I have seen, no hard science. But it's pretty spot on in the patients I see. If you want to know your testosterone level the only 'true' way is to do a blood test.

The algorithm is based on this pant size (33% information from the elevated aromatase levels) and based on age as most men lose about a percent a year of testosterone after the age of 30 to surmise this formula. I will say that age is probably pretty insignificant in the big scheme of things as you will see below.

I will also say that if you aren't familiar with pant size increase, one pant size equates to about 20 pounds overweight. So you can use the formula as for each 20 pounds overweight = 33%, or each pant size = 33%

We will call this a 'point system' as well. Testosterone in the blood is usually measured in the laboratory as 'ng/dL' but we will just use a whole number and call it a point just for simplicity or your T-score which can range from this lab in the example below from 250-1100.

TESTOSTERONE, FREE,BIO AND TOTAL, LC/MS/MS TESTOSTERONE, TOTAL, LC/MS/MS	707	250-1100 ng/dL

Formula:

Age in years over 30 x 1% + 33% for each pant size over your ideal.

So if you are man who is 40 years old that's 40 years-30 years= 10 years x 1% (for each year) = total 10% decline so if maximum is 1100 (most testosterone ranges from 250-1100) so just by age you can subtract 120. Now your score is 980. Then for each pant size up (lets assume 20 pounds for each additional pant size) lets say you are 40 pounds over weight now you have you are down 66% (33% x 2) which is another minus 726 points (or 66% 0f 1100). So if you are a man, 40 years old with and extra 40 lbs. your testosterone is probably 1100-120-726= 254. Your score is probably around 254! Pretty cool huh? You do the math. How old are you and how overweight are you?

And of course, I'll say again, while this is kind of cool and works pretty darn close most of the time, I do recommend you get your levels checked with a blood test, as many other factors can lower your levels to as mentioned above.

If you aren't a math nerd or hate to do math like a lot of us I have created a little table based on your age and how overweight you are to help you make a quick estimate.

Of course, you can't go into the negative but you can be non-detectable on assay so if you are more than 60 pounds overweight and 70 or 80 years old your levels will be pretty darn low unless you have some other compensation from the adrenal glands going on which commonly does happen.

But to be smart about things you also need several other hormones checked too. Here is the list I recommend.

[]Testosterone (free and total)
[]Estradiol/Estrone (Estrogens)
[]Progesterone
[] DHT (Dihydrotestosterone)
[]SHBG (Sex Hormone Binding Globulin)
[]FSH/LH
[]Insulin
[]TSH (Pituitary Thyroid Stimulating Hormone)
[]Free T3 (Thyroid)
[]PSA (Prostate Specific Antigen)
[]CBC (Complete Blood Count)

1. Testosterone – Free and total, best done in the early a.m. Free testosterone is the amount of testosterone unbound, free and available to the tissues.
2. Estradiol and Estrone – These levels are important for tracking estrogen conversion through aromatase.
3. Progesterone – A precursor hormone for all other sex steroid hormones, important for sleep in both men and women and to balance out estrogen to prevent prostate cancer (and breast cancer in women)
4. Dihydrotestosterone – End point sex steroid hormone from testosterone that if too high can cause prostate enlargement and male pattern hair loss (think Mr. Clean… LOL), acne and ear hair (ewe gross…
5. SHBG – Sex Hormone Binding Globulin, the little carrier proteins that carry your testosterone around (think free or total testosterone), can be low if you don't consume enough protein as it is made out of protein.

6. FSH/LH – Pituitary or brain stimulating hormones often used to diagnose primary or secondary testosterone deficiency. Used by hormone doctors to make sure nothing more serious is wrong especially in younger patients.

7. Insulin – Blood sugar/glucose storage hormone if elevated often used in the diagnosis of insulin resistance, metabolic syndrome ... precursors to diabetes which are all a risk of low T.

8. Thyroid – Master of metabolism and often affected by testosterone issues. Can cause weight gain and fatigue. You don't want to miss a low thyroid, as you might not think testosterone therapy is working to help you feel better if you have missed a low thyroid.

9. PSA – Prostate Specific Antigen used for diagnosing prostate issues including cancer. Good to have as a baseline. Although low T and high estrogens are a risk factor for prostate cancer, it's still good to know where you stand.

10. CBC – Sometimes testosterone therapy if the estrogen conversion is not closely monitored can cause thickening of the red blood cells, which may cause blood pressure issues, lung or heart issues.

These comprehensive tests will also help you to know if your testosterone clinic is educated on all the aspects of testosterone. If they only check testosterone they clearly don't understand about estrogen conversion and the risks. You need some estrogen to keep men empathetic and help with bone density, skin youth, cardiovascular protection and memory. To much estrogen and you get man boobs, prostate issues and impotence.

Misdiagnosed thyroid issues and insulin issues can make testosterone therapy seem ineffective. Make sure you ask for all of these tests.

The REAL Reason You Are Feeling Physically, Mentally & Sexually Tapped Out...

If you are not feeling like the man you once were, testosterone – or the lack thereof – is the most likely culprit.

Testosterone is responsible for sustaining your mental focus, energy, metabolism, muscle mass, fat levels, and sex drive.

As a man, your natural hormones, specifically your testosterone levels, begin to decline in your mid-20s. Hormone imbalance symptoms normally show up before or during your mid-30s.

This low testosterone condition is also called andropause, or the "male menopause", and is responsible for all the symptoms you've been feeling (as well as many more that will emerge over time.) The good news is you can restore your vitality and reduce the symptoms of andropause by balancing your hormone levels.

You may hear it called "Testosterone Replacement Therapy", however I don't believe that you are 'replacing' anything but rather supplementing your levels in a natural way. In fact, some wives are worried about their husbands getting 'roid rage' or irritable. What I tell them is that there is a range (250 to 1100) and we test levels to keep them in the natural therapeutic youthful ranges – up to at least 1000 and never greater than 1400 - because at higher levels you can get anger issues and pituitary or brain suppression of your own natural testosterone, in addition to the many of the other side effects associated with too much testosterone. Yes, too much of anything is not a good thing. And the more testosterone you have the more potential conversion to estrogen and estrogen side effects. I will discuss the side effects of too much estrogen in more detail later.

You don't have to go through this alone. There is a solution. You can get your life back ... more strength, more stamina, and more vitality than ever before!
It's time for a BIG change:

- ☐ No more feeling exhausted
- ☐ No more aches and pains
- ☐ No more irritability, sadness, or moodiness
- ☐ No more lowered or decreased sex drive or fears of failing in the bedroom
- ☐ No more restless nights because of poor sleep
- ☐ No more problems focusing

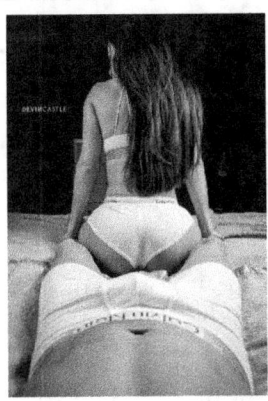

CHAPTER 2 - I'M TOO EMBARRASSED

"I'm Too Embarrassed...Could Hormone Replacement Really Be For Me?"

In the past, we've had clients say, "Oh, I could never do something like that. It all seems too embarrassing."

Isn't it more embarrassing to not perform in the bedroom like you know you used to? Isn't it more embarrassing to gain weight in all the wrong places and not like the way you look? Isn't it more embarrassing to not have the stamina you used to? Isn't it more embarrassing when you are passed over for opportunities and job advancements by younger men? Isn't it more embarrassing to lose your energy and drive? I tell my patients that libido is the last thing to go and it's not a matter of your "manhood" or that something is wrong... it's just simply a choice to maximize what mother nature designed you to have. It's so easy to get tested and you can do it privately. If you are concerned that someone might know your score (and now they might when that algorithm hits mainstream) then do something now to get your testosterone back to youthful levels.

The bottom line: isn't it more embarrassing when other guys always seem to have the competitive edge over you while you just settle for declining testosterone levels? Isn't it more embarrassing that your family doesn't get the wildfire, motivated, spit-fire energetic husband and father that they could have?

Will it be more embarrassing when you get diabetes (as low T is a risk for insulin resistance) and lose a toe or foot? Will it be more embarrassing if you get prostate cancer (another risk factor for low T) and they do surgery or radiation and you get nerve damage as a complication and then cannot have an erection or you become incontinent?

Will it be more embarrassing if you gain a lot of weight and feel tired and sluggish?

Ask yourself what your real fear is? Is it that you are not going to be considered 'man enough' if your T is low?

Consider this. All our buddies are probably getting tested and you probably don't even know. Testing is done confidentially. In fact medical providers are required by federal law not to discuss your medical information. You can get tested and at least know that you have normal levels or you don't. Why stay in the dark? Seriously???

What are you afraid of? Knowledge is power. Power to help you maximize your health, stave of aging (which is just hormone decline) and the power to look, feel and think at your most optimum level.

You are a 'rock star' and you deserve to feel like one!

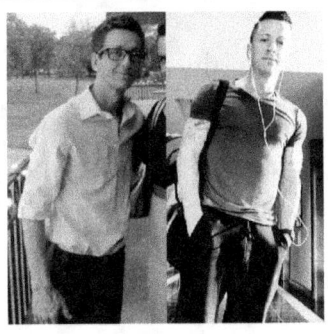

CHAPTER 3 - IS IT SAFE?

There is so much fear in medicine. Doctors have been operating out of fear for so long even the doctors don't know what to believe anymore. Let's talk about the great testosterone myth that scares everyone including doctors. In fact it is almost single-handedly the main reason that doctors are not only afraid of prescribing testosterone, but even when they do prescribe it, it may only treat men to suboptimal levels. The truth is that risk of cancer and disease is increased with low T and there is a lot of research to back that up. Lets talk about how all the fear and myth got started. What is the myth?

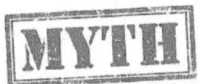

TESTOSTERONE CAUSES PROSTATE
CANCER

It has long been believed that low testosterone levels could help protect a man from developing prostate cancer. Furthermore, many doctors believed that giving a man with undetected prostate cancer Testosterone Replacement Therapy would ultimately worsen his condition. It was not until recently that many doctors began to see these beliefs for the myths that they are.

While it was medically proven a long time ago that low testosterone levels actually increase the risk of a man developing prostate cancer, it can take a long time to expel a widely accepted myth such as the one discussed above.

If you are struggling to accept the fact that low T-levels can increase your chances of developing prostate cancer, take a moment to consider the research of Dr. Abraham Morgentaler. As part of his research Dr. Morgentaler looked at every study ever published on the topic of prostate cancer and hormone levels. Additionally, Dr. Morgentaler performed several studies of his own. Through this research he established several key facts:

- Low testosterone levels do not protect against prostate cancer. In fact, they can increase your risk.
- High levels of testosterone in the blood do not increase your chances of developing prostate cancer.

The use of Testosterone Replacement Therapy did not increase the risk of developing prostate cancer, even in men with a high risk of developing this cancer.

Still not ready to abandon the myth that high testosterone levels can increase your risk of prostate cancer? Consider this: Prostate cancer rarely affects men in their 20's; however, this is when men experience a natural height in their testosterone production. If high testosterone levels resulted in a higher risk of prostate cancer, men would be at a higher risk of developing this disease in their youth rather than as they age.

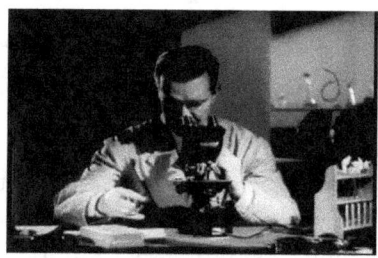

Wondering where this wide spread myth started? Well you may be surprised to learn that this myth started as the result of a 1941 study conducted by Dr. Higgins. This study consisted of only **three** men, but only reported on the findings of two of them. To make matters worse, one of the men included in the study had been previously castrated.

When challenging this controversial study, many doctors will also refer to another old study published in 1981, which backed up the findings of Dr. Higgins. While this study did make use of more participants, only four of the men who participated in the study had not received some type of prior hormone treatment. These treatments included castration and estrogen. Furthermore, all four of these men responded positively to the use of Testosterone Therapy.

At the conclusion of his research, Dr. Morgentaler found that no published studies to date could demonstrate a direct relationship between high testosterone levels and an increased risk of prostate cancer.

In 2006, Dr. Morgentaler teamed up with Dr. Rhoden to conduct another study on the topic. The findings of this study were concurrent with his previous studies, ultimately showing that men with lower testosterone levels were at a higher risk of developing prostate cancer. Studies conducted by other doctors all over the world have continuously backed up these findings. Unfortunately, despite the overwhelming medical facts, there are still many patients and doctors who hold onto the old myth that TRT can increase the risk of prostate cancer. Through the use of successful therapy and public education we hope to change that in the near future.

The question that I ask patients to consider is if testosterone increased your risk of prostate cancer or fueled prostate cancer, then why don't we seen teenage boys with prostate cancer when their levels are the highest?

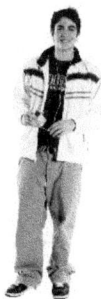

**How Many Teenage Boys
Do You Know
With
Prostate Cancer?**

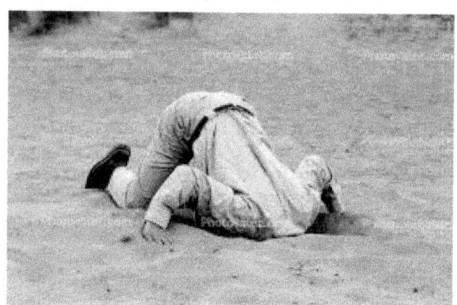

CHAPTER 4 - IS THERE A RISK IF I DO NOTHING?

Have you ever asked yourself what "aging" really is? Aging is the decline of hormones that normally maintain youthful processes. Testosterone is an anabolic steroid, which promotes growth and frankly, if you are not growing, you are dying!

Testosterone is a 19-carbon steroid hormone produced primarily by the Leydig cells of the testes (in men) and the ovaries (in women). Smaller amounts are produced in the adrenal glands of both sexes. Yes, men and women both make and have testosterone.

In men, approximately seven mg of testosterone is produced each day, and blood levels range between 250 and 1200 ng/dL (10-28 nmol/L).

Testosterone levels are high in young men, but plummet as they age. Despite compelling findings of efficacy, conventional doctors still question the value of testosterone replacement in maturing men. This oversight is causing needless heart attacks and strokes.

Having low testosterone can increase your risk of not only prostate cancer as previously discussed but also the risk of:
-excess abdominal fat
-insulin resistance
-diabetes
-atherosclerosis (hardening of the arteries... heart and brain artery disease)
-memory loss

How can this all be? A critically important role of testosterone is to enable HDL (good cholesterol) to remove excess cholesterol from the arterial wall and transport it to the liver for disposal. This effect of enhancing HDL is termed "reverse cholesterol transport" and is vital to preventing arterial occlusion.

One of my biggest frustrations from the traditional medicine hamster wheel is that cardiologists routinely prescribe statin drugs to lower LDL, a lipoprotein that transports cholesterol from the liver to the arteries. These same doctors, however, fail to maintain sufficient testosterone levels in their patients to enable HDL to remove cholesterol buildup in the arteries. This is one reason why statin drugs have not always been shown to work in older men, who require functional HDL to keep arterial linings free of excess cholesterol.

Numerous studies document the vital role that testosterone plays in maintaining youthful metabolic processes throughout the body. A large new study confirms the deadly impact of low testosterone in older men.

What's scary are clinical trials designed by doctors who have no idea how to achieve youthful hormone levels. Men who enroll in these studies are subjected to lethal dangers because testosterone and estrogen blood levels are not properly balanced.

Cells throughout a man's body are laden with receptor sites that are activated by the hormone testosterone. When testosterone is available to bind to these receptor sites good things happen, such as elevated mood and improved cognition in response to plentiful testosterone being available to the brain.

Be it muscle, bone, vascular, or nerve tissue, testosterone provides critical command signals for your cells to behave in a youthful manner. As testosterone levels diminish, degenerative processes set in.

Of considerable interest is the relationship between testosterone blood levels and cardiovascular events such as heart attack and stroke. In a revealing new study, researchers identified 2,416 men (aged 69-81 years) who were not on any kind of testosterone-affecting treatment. These men were subjected to a battery of blood tests that included total testosterone and estradiol (estrogen).

The first observation was that men with increasing levels of testosterone had a decreased prevalence of diabetes, hypertension, and body fat mass.

Testosterone and Stroke Risk
One way to evaluate one's risk for a stroke is to undergo an ultrasound test to measure carotid artery thickness. When excess occlusion is detected, a risky surgical procedure (carotid endarterectomy) is performed to restore blood flow to the brain.

In a study published by the American Heart Association in April 2004, ultrasounds were used to measure the carotid intima-media thickness in 195 independently-living elderly men in 1996 and again in 2000. The researchers also measured blood levels of free testosterone in these men.

The results showed that men with low testosterone had a 3.57 times greater progression of carotid intima-media thickening than those with higher testosterone levels which can lead to a stroke!

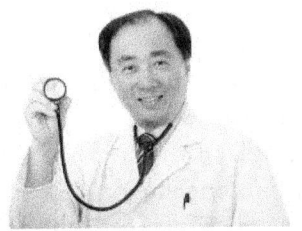

CHAPTER 5 - CAN ANY DOCTOR TREAT LOW TESTOSTERONE?

Yes, any medical doctor can test your blood, diagnose, and treat your low T. There are low T clinics popping up all over the place. Body builders have been experimenting with testosterone therapy for years and we have learned a lot from them. Traditional medicine, however, has turned a blind eye to the knowledge that this fitness culture has brought to light.

We know a few things from the mistakes that body builders have made:
-Don't go too high with levels. High levels can cause 'roid rage', shrink your testicles, suppress your natural testosterone, and cause your breasts to enlarge (man boobs.)
-Don't take testosterone orally (by mouth.) It must go through the liver in what is called first-pass metabolism. Testosterone taken orally can essentially "blow out the liver", causing liver damage and inflammation.
-There are many different forms of testosterone. Some are safer while others have more side effects (more of a discussion than we have time for here.)

One of the biggest issues with testosterone therapy is that with the widespread use and marketing of "Low T", clinics are popping up that are not taking into account all the hormones that affect and interact with testosterone, most remarkably ESTROGEN. Without monitoring estrogen you put a man at great risk.

The conversion of testosterone to estrogen through aromatase is an easy process to track and to responsibly treat, but rarely addressed by these fly-by-night testosterone clinics and even well-meaning primary care physicians and urologists.

When you are making your choice to get therapy make sure you do your homework and work with a practitioner who understands the relationship between all of the steroid hormones and estrogen. You should have testing to check estrogen levels, thyroid, adrenal hormones, complete blood count (for red blood cells, white blood cells and platelets), and PSA (prostate specific antigen-test for prostate cancer) to get a comprehensive look at all of your hormones. It is important that your estrogen levels are kept within a certain range (too high or too low can cause complications), blood count is within normal range (testosterone can increase red blood cells), and no active prostate cancer is present (because estrogen conversion from testosterone may be an issues.)

The biggest issue for men undergoing testosterone therapy occurs with the conversion to estrogen. A certain form of estrogen called estrone can cause all the issues or problematic side effects that we see with testosterone therapy (or with estrogen therapy in women.) This estrogen can be proliferative and cause prostate enlargement (proliferation) and/or cancer.

This is why we often prescribe estrogen blockers to keep the estrogen conversion from becoming a problem.

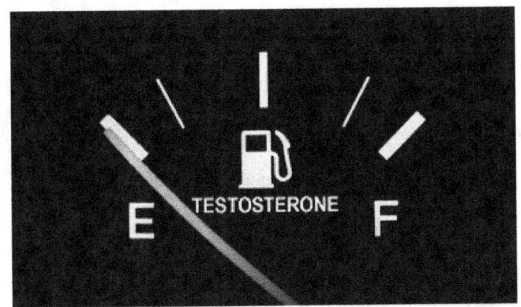

CHAPTER 6 - MY "T" IS LOW... NOW WHAT?

What are Your Options for Replacement?

If your levels are indeed low, there are a number of synthetic and bio-identical (I only recommend bio-identical because they are the same as your own body's production) testosterone products on the market. There is also DHEA, which is the most abundant androgen precursor prohormone in the human body, meaning that it is the largest raw material your body uses to produce other vital hormones, including testosterone in men. The first thing to understand about testosterone replacement is that oral testosterone (pills taken by mouth) doesn't really work because it is broken down so quickly by the liver. The solution to this problem involves patches, gels, pellets, troches and shots. Here are the different options further defined:

If you've done any research on low testosterone treatment options, you've probably come across a wide variety of recommendations. Some will tell you that pellets are the best form of treatment. Other people will swear by topicals.

I have specific practices in place based on recommendations by the Endocrine Society and my own experience over the past 16 years in practice.

Injections

This regimen consists of weekly or bi-weekly injections of testosterone cypionate usually in 100 or 200 mg/cc of injectable solution.

I recommend weekly injections of testosterone to keep your levels optimal - not too high, not too low. These weekly injections also allow for the use of the lowest effective dose, which decreases the potential for side effects. These intramuscular injections go deep into the muscle and dissolve over time. The amount of time it takes for the injection to dissolve depends on the half-life of the testosterone cypionate, which is about 8 days. I've found that injections cause your numbers to go up in the first 48 hours, but within 8 days the amount of medicine in your body reduces by half. That's why I do weekly injections - an injection on day 7 gets your numbers back up where they need to be. Your levels will still fluctuate with testosterone injections, but the fluctuations will be much less than other low testosterone treatment options.

Topicals (Creams, Gels, and Patches)

While we recognize that men respond most favorably to injection therapy, some patients are not candidates for traditional testosterone replacement and may benefit from topical testosterone gel preparations (AndroGel, Testim, Axiron, Fortesta.) This is the only low testosterone treatment option that requires a daily dosage. While application is simple, be aware there are side effects. And even though topicals seem like a great solution because you don't have to make weekly visits to the clinic, they do have some issues.

First, topicals be transferred from your skin on to the skin of other people, like your wife or your kids. You don't want to be transmitting this hormone to people who don't need it. Second, topicals can be very expensive because insurance usually doesn't cover them. Third, some men find that topicals irritate their skin. If you already experience skin problems, topicals might not be a great solution for you. Finally, and this is the biggest issue, topicals tend to have a high failure rate. Somewhere between 30-40% of men cannot absorb enough of the topicals through their skin to improve their testosterone levels.

This is why out of all the low testosterone treatment options I recommend injections. Not only do they have a higher success rate, but they have fewer drawbacks when compared to topicals.

Pellets

Another one of the popular low testosterone treatment options is the testosterone pellets. Pellets are compounded testosterone medications that are surgically implanted under your skin. The pellets release the medication over a period of months.

These pellets are inserted two to three times a year and a great option if you travel a lot. The expense over time is about the same as injections.

The only concern with pellets is the dip in testosterone levels as they near replacement time. However, the upside to pellets is the convenience and the fact that estrogen blockers can be combined into the pellets so you don't have to take additional tablets along with your injections.

Troches

Troches are dissolvable tablets that are placed under the tongue and dissolve in about 3-5 minutes. This option is a good alternative for those who are fearful of needles, aren't a good candidate for creams or gels, or do not want pellets. Troches can also have estrogen blockers or DHT blockers compounded into them.

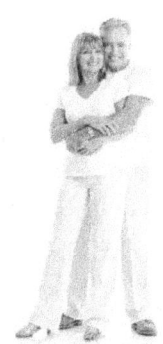

CHAPTER 7 - NATURAL OPTIONS FOR INCREASING "T"

Lose Weight

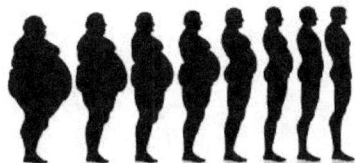

This is a tricky one. Oftentimes it's hard to lose weight if your testosterone is low and you may opt for testosterone therapy to make weight loss easier. The fact remains though, if you are overweight, shedding the excess pounds may increase your testosterone levels, according to research presented at the Endocrine Society's 2012 meeting. Overweight men are more likely to have low testosterone levels to begin with, so this is an important trick to increase your body's testosterone production when you need it most.

If you are serious about losing weight, it is imperative that you strictly limit the amount of processed sugar in your diet, as evidence is mounting that excess sugar, fructose in particular, is the primary driving factor in the obesity epidemic. Cutting soda from your diet is essential, as is limiting fructose found in processed foods, fruit juice, excessive fruit and so-called "healthy" sweeteners derived from stevia or agave.

Ideally you should keep your total fructose consumption below 25 grams per day and this includes fruits. This is especially true if you are insulin-resistant, overweight, have high blood pressure, and/or diabetic.

Refined carbohydrates like breakfast cereals, bagels, waffles, pretzels, and most other processed foods quickly break down to sugar, increase your insulin levels, and cause insulin resistance, which is the number one underlying factor of nearly every chronic disease and condition known to man, including weight gain.

Exercise:

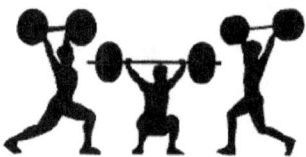

Strength training with weights

In addition to peak fitness, strength training is also known to boost testosterone levels, provided your intensity level is sufficient. When strength training to boost testosterone you will want to increase the weight and lower your number of reps, focusing on exercises that work a large number of muscles, such as dead lifts or squats.

You can "turbo-charge" your weight training by going slower. By slowing down your movement, you are actually turning it into a high-intensity exercise. Super slow movement allows your muscle, at the microscopic level, to access the maximum number of cross-bridges between the protein filaments that produce movement in the muscle.

High-intensity exercise like Peak Fitness (especially when combined with intermittent fasting) and short, intense exercise have been shown to boost testosterone.

Short, intense exercise has a proven positive effect on increasing testosterone levels while also preventing its decline. That's unlike aerobics or prolonged moderate exercise, which have shown to have negative or no effect on testosterone levels. Intermittent fasting boosts testosterone by increasing the expression of satiety hormones including insulin, leptin, adiponectin, glucagon-like peptide-1 (GLP-1), cholecystokinin (CKK) and melanocortins, all of which are known to potentiate healthy testosterone actions, increase libido, and prevent age-related testosterone decline.

Having a whey protein meal after exercise can further enhance the satiety/testosterone-boosting impact (hunger hormones cause the opposite effect on your testosterone and libido.)

Here's a summary of what a typical high-intensity Peak Fitness routine might look like:

Warm up for three minutes
Exercise as hard and fast as you can for 30 seconds. You should feel like you couldn't possibly go on another few seconds.
Recover at a slow to moderate pace for 90 seconds.
Repeat the high intensity exercise and recovery 7 more times.

As you can see, the entire workout is only 20 minutes. 20 minutes! That really is a beautiful thing. And within those 20 minutes, 75% of that time is warming up, recovering or cooling down. You are really only working out intensely for four minutes. It's hard to believe if you have never done this before that you can actually benefit from only four minutes of exercise. It is that simple.

As long as you are pushing yourself as hard as you can for 30 seconds, you can use virtually any type of equipment or none at all for this workout - an elliptical machine, a treadmill, swimming, or even sprinting outdoors, although you will need to do this very carefully as to avoid injury. Always be sure to stretch properly and start slowly to avoid injury. Begin with two or three repetitions and work your way up, and don't expect to do all eight repetitions the first time you try this, especially if you are out of shape.

Supplements

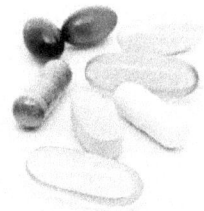

ZINC

The mineral zinc is important for testosterone production and supplementing your diet for as little as six weeks has been shown to cause a marked improvement in testosterone among men with low levels. Similarly, research has shown that restricting dietary sources of zinc leads to a significant decrease in testosterone, while zinc supplementation not only increases testosterone, it even protects men from exercised-induced reductions in testosterone levels.

It's estimated that up to 45% of adults over the age of 60 may have lower than recommended zinc intakes; even when dietary supplements were added in, an estimated 20-25% of older adults still had inadequate zinc intakes.

Your diet is the best source of zinc. Along with protein-rich foods like meats and fish, other good dietary sources of zinc include raw milk, raw cheese, beans, and yogurt or kefir made from raw milk. It can be difficult to obtain enough dietary zinc for vegetarians and meat-eaters alike, largely because of conventional farming methods which rely heavily on chemical fertilizers and pesticides. These chemicals deplete the soil of nutrients - like zinc that must be absorbed by plants in order to be passed on to you.

In many cases, you may further deplete the nutrients in your food by the way you prepare it. Cooking, particularly overcooking, most foods will drastically reduce the levels of nutrients such as zinc. If you decide to use a zinc supplement, stick to a dosage of less than 40 mg a day, as this is the recommended adult upper limit. Taking too much zinc can interfere with your body's ability to absorb other minerals, especially copper, and may cause nausea as a side effect.

Optimize Your Vitamin D Levels

Vitamin D increases levels of testosterone. In one study, overweight men who were given vitamin D supplements had a significant increase in testosterone levels after one year.

Vitamin D deficiency is currently at epidemic proportions in the United States and many other regions around the world, largely because people do not spend enough time in the sun to facilitate the important process of vitamin D production.

So the first step to ensuring you are receiving all the benefits of vitamin D is to find out what your levels are using a 25(OH)D test, also called 25-hydroxyvitamin D.

A few years back, the recommended level was between 40 to 60 nanograms per milliliter (ng/ml), but more recently the optimal vitamin D level has been raised to 70-80 ng/ml.

To get your levels into the healthy range, sun exposure is the BEST way to optimize your vitamin D levels; exposing a large amount of your skin until it turns the lightest shade of pink, as near to solar noon as possible, is typically necessary to achieve adequate vitamin D production. If sun exposure is not an option, a safe tanning bed (with electronic ballasts rather than magnetic ballasts, to avoid unnecessary exposure to EMF fields) can be used.

As a last resort, a vitamin D3 supplement can be taken orally, but research suggests the average adult needs to take 10,000 IU's of vitamin D per day in order to elevate their levels above 40 ng/ml, which is the absolute minimum for disease prevention.

Reduce Stress

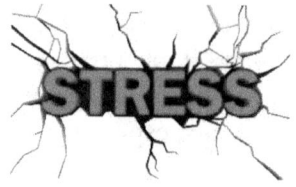

When you are under a lot of stress, your body releases high levels of the stress hormone cortisol. This hormone actually blocks the effects of testosterone, presumably because, from a biological standpoint, testosterone-associated behaviors (i.e., mating, competing, aggression) may have lowered your chances of survival in an emergency (hence, the "fight or flight" response is dominant, courtesy of cortisol.)

In the modern world, chronic stress, and subsequently elevated levels of cortisol, could mean that testosterone's effects are blocked in the long term, which is what you want to avoid.

Some common stress-reduction tools with a high success rate include prayer, meditation, laughter, and yoga, for example. Learning relaxation skills, such as deep breathing and positive visualization - the "language" of the subconscious – will also help with stress reduction. When you create a visual image of how you'd like to feel, your subconscious will understand and begin to help you by making the needed biochemical and neurological changes.

Stress can also be in the form of toxins (alcohol is the main one), pesticides, chemicals in plastics and environmental as well as through Leaky gut and food triggers.

We recommend that you learn more about leaky gut and food sensitivity testing (IgG) and talk to a health coach about a detox plan for your liver.

Eat Healthy Fats

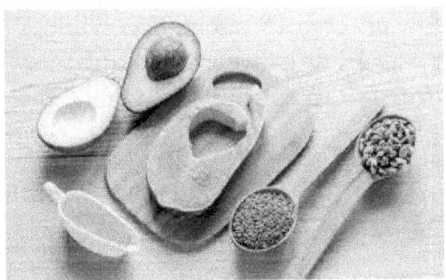

By healthy, this means not only mono- and polyunsaturated fats, like that found in avocadoes and nuts, but also saturated fats, as these are essential for building testosterone. Research shows that a diet with less than 40% of energy as fat (that mainly comes from animal sources, i.e. saturated) can lead to a decrease in testosterone levels.
Most experts agree that the ideal diet includes somewhere between 50-70 % fat.

It's important to understand that your body requires saturated fats from animal and vegetable sources (such as meat, dairy, certain oils, and tropical plants like coconut) for optimal functioning, and if you neglect this important food group in favor of sugar, grains, and other starchy carbs, your health and weight are almost guaranteed to suffer.

Branch Chain Amino Acids (BCAA's) from Foods Like Whey Protein

Research suggests that BCAA's result in higher testosterone levels, particularly when taken along with resistance training. While BCAA's are available in supplement form, you'll find the highest concentrations of BCAA's like leucine in dairy products, especially quality cheeses and whey protein.

Even when getting leucine from your natural food supply, it's often wasted or used as a building block instead of an anabolic agent. So to create the correct anabolic environment you need to boost leucine consumption way beyond mere maintenance levels.

That said, keep in mind that using leucine as a free form amino acid can be highly counterproductive because when free form amino acids are artificially administrated, they rapidly enter your circulation while disrupting insulin function, impairing your body's glycemic control. Food-based leucine is really the ideal form to maximize the benefits to your muscles without the added side effects.

Have your food allergies/sensitivities checked

Leaky gut issues can lead to inflammation in the gut. Certain foods may trigger more inflammation which can lead to excess cortisol production. Avoiding these foods can help your testosterone levels.

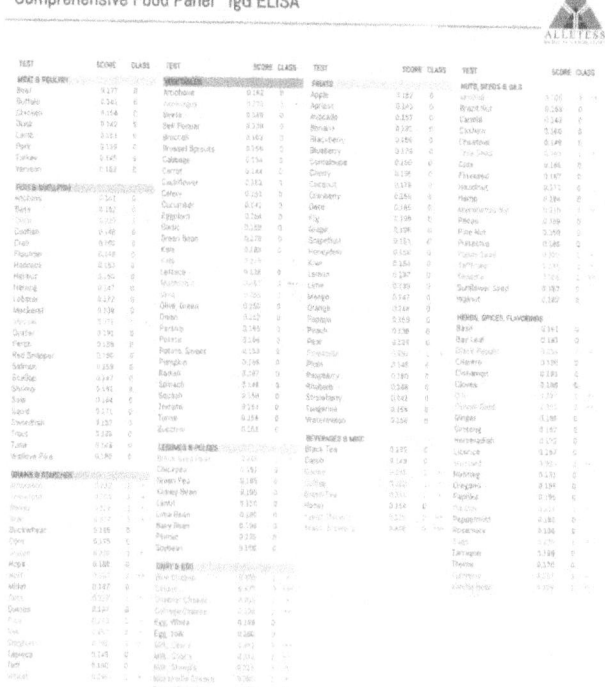

Comprehensive Food Panel IgG ELISA

Get adequate sleep

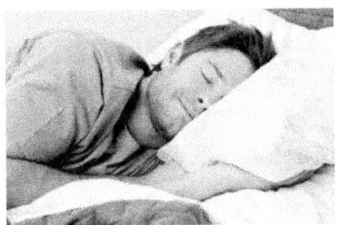

Again this is one symptom that can stem from low testosterone. Testosterone therapy may help you sleep better, but if you are a technology junkie, turn off the electronics and invest in the practice of good sleep hygiene.

Have more sex

Frequent sex can actually stimulate the testicles to make more testosterone.

Detox and Methylation

Supplements that help detox the body like methyl-folate can help clear abnormal accumulations of estrogen and boost testosterone.

Avoid Alcohol

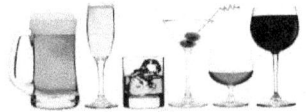

Alcohol is a toxin that can affect the liver and prevent it from proper detoxification and methylation.

All of the above should be combined in an overall health program.

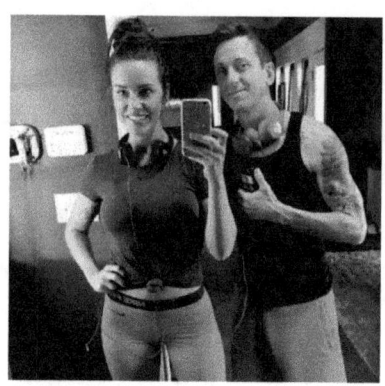

CHAPTER 8 - SUMMARY

There is no reason to be afraid of testosterone therapy as long as it is done with natural bio-identical testosterone or other hormones as indicated, frequent testing is performed to monitor for safety, and it is done as a comprehensive overall wellness approach for anti-aging and health.

Do your homework and find experts who are going to help you understand all aspects of your therapy.

Call your provider if you experience any adverse affects. Monitor your blood pressure regularly and educate and empower yourself in all aspects of your therapy.

If you want to look and feel your best and regain your youth and health while pursuing anti-aging and optimal health then testosterone therapy may just be an option for you.

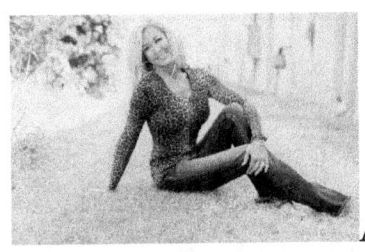

ABOUT THE AUTHOR

Dr. Tammy has spent many years cultivating a culture of accountability in patients. She has motivated and mentored many in the ways of improving their own health, one healthy decision at a time. Born and raised in a small town in Arkansas, she pursued her training all throughout the U.S. and is grounded and in tune with the simple to the sophisticated when it comes to educating her patients. Her extensive work and educational background lends to her non-traditional physician approach. She went beyond attaining a bachelor's degree in biology to pursing her master's degree in public health. While doing this, she began teaching and discovered a passion for educating as a means to spawn greatness and discovery in others. She then attended 4 years of medical school at Kansas City University of Medicine and Biosciences, plus an additional year at Truman Medical Center as a Pathology Fellow, teaching and learning about the basics of human processes. Her goal was to integrate all these experiences so she could be the best family physician and health educator-mentor possible. She did her residency in Tallahassee, Florida. She is currently a board-certified family practice physician licensed to practice in the state of Arkansas.

She has done award-winning research in multiple areas, including education, cancer, and biologic hormone processes. She has focused additional emphasis on programs promoting wellness and preventive care. She offers her patients a unique approach to medicine by bringing an extensive education, a desire to help others, and a genuine desire to make the medical experience a positive one for all patients. She empowers patients to take charge of their own wellbeing and health through the balance of hormones, stress reduction, detox, supplements, and fitness. Oh, and she brings a BIG SMILE! Those who know her will confirm she loves enlightening, educating, and empowering others to pursue healthy lifestyles. She has spent the past few years transforming into everything she recommends. She definitely practices what she preaches!

Testimonials

"After six years of driving a semi-truck all over this great country I had quite frankly become fat as hell and lazy. My old lady was complaining, my kids were complaining, I think my dog would've complained if he could've. I decided to get off of my ass and get in shape. After a year steady in the gym I was feeling better about myself but I was still fat, still out of shape, no miracle man for sure. After doing some research I decided to have my testosterone levels checked. Wow 173, I had no idea and normal is at least 800 and 1000-1200 is ideal. I started my regimen a week later and it's now been four months. In four months I've lost more weight, gained more strength, and begun to see more muscle develop " in my legs, chest and arms than in a whole year previously! You guys have truly helped me to become a better husband and dad."-Tony H.

"I was skeptical, hell I am the biggest skeptic you'll ever meet, but I gotta give it to Better Living Rx, they do what they say they are gonna do. I received my testosterone in a timely manner and have loved the results. Not gonna lie and tell you I'm having sex everyday cause I ain't...I work for a living and I'm tired at night. But then again, my old lady ain't complaining one bit!" – Patrick W.

"Literally stopping the aging process and turning back your body's clock to a younger, fresher, more energized you. I feel stronger. I'm sleeping better and I've lost twenty pounds in less than three months. I couldn't be more satisfied.
–Richard P.

"Never thought I'd have the nerve to give myself a shot in the butt or anywhere for that matter, but once I saw the video I gave it a try and I was surprised how easy it was. I'm now into my fifth month of the regimen and I'm feeling great, and the injections are easy and pretty much painless. Thanks for making this available without all of the hassles of driving across town to wait in an office!" –George H.

"I feel like if there is a fountain of youth you guys may have discovered it! I feel great. In fact, I haven't felt this good since I was a senior in
high school having the time of my life on the football field. I'm stronger, have more energy and feel better than ever." -Sam S.

"My golf score has improved. I'm swinging harder. Hitting the ball farther, and when I get home I'm ready to do more. I'd say what you offered is exactly what I needed." -Russ S.

"So grateful to finally lose that belly fat and feel younger and better. I lost 30 pounds in three months with eating better and exercising and testosterone therapy. I am eating better and have regained focus on taking care of myself again."
-Frank S.

Frank

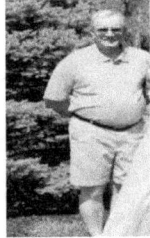 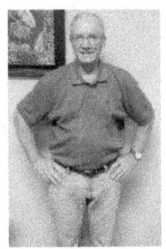

Before   **3 months**

"Just wanted to say thank you for helping me. You've helped give me life again and I'm so thankful. You are truly special." -Jeremy J.

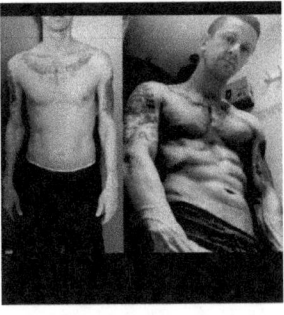

www.ingramcontent.com/pod-product-compliance
Lightning Source LLC
Chambersburg PA
CBHW072139290526
45789CB00013B/1573